Copyright 2023

All right reserved. No part of this book should be reproduced without express permission of the author.

Reproduction of all or any part of this book is punishable under relevant law.

Table of Contents

A migraine is a headache that can cause severe throbbing pain or a pulsing sensation, usually on one side of the head. It's often accompanied by nausea, vomiting, and extreme sensitivity to light and sound. Migraine attacks can last for hours to days, and the pain can be so severe that it interferes with your daily activities.

For some people, a warning symptom known as an aura occurs before or with the headache. An aura can include visual disturbances, such as flashes of light or blind spots, or other disturbances, such as tingling on one side of the face or in an arm or leg and difficulty speaking.

Medications can help prevent some migraines and make them less painful. The right medicines, combined with self-help remedies and lifestyle changes, might help.

1. Oatmeal Muffins

Prep Time: 15 Minutes

Cook Time: 20 Minutes

Servings: 12

Ingredients

- 1¼ cups rolled oats
- 1¼ cups all purpose flour
- 2 teaspoons baking powder
- ½ teaspoon baking soda
- ½ teaspoon cinnamon
- ½ teaspoon kosher salt
- ½ cup gently packed light brown sugar
- ⅓ cup apple sauce
- 1 large egg
- ½ cup vegetable oil

- ¾ cup milk of choice
- 1 teaspoon vanilla extract
- 1½ cups fresh, blackberries, cut in small pieces
- 1½ tablespoons white sugar

Instructions

1. Preheat oven to 425 degrees F. In a medium bowl, combine the dry ingredients - rolled oats (NOT quick cooking/instant/steel cut), flour, baking powder, baking soda, cinnamon, and ½ teaspoon salt. Stir to combine. In a separate large bowl, combine the sugar, apple sauce, egg, vegetable oil, milk, vanilla,. Mix until thoroughly combined and smooth. Add the flour mixture to the wet ingredients, stirring till just incorporated. Do not overmix.

2. Taste the blackberries, if sweet, no extra sugar is needed. If a bit tart, stir them with 1 ½ tablespoons of white sugar, then gently fold into the batter till just mixed.

3. Prepare a muffin pan with paper cups or grease the pan well. Fill the batter, almost to the top of the

cups or pan. Sprinkle the tops with extra white sugar and rolled oats, if desired.

4. Bake at 425 degrees F for 5 minutes, then reduce the heat to 350 degrees F without removing the muffins. Bake another 15-17 minutes until cooked through. Allow the muffins to cool in the pan for about 5 minutes then remove to continue to cool on a wire rack. If you eat them while still hot, they'll be more crumbly!

5. My oven is recently calibrated and these took exactly 20 minutes to be done. It's better to go low on the cooking time. If cooked too much, these will be more crumbly.

6. Sub 1 egg with your favorite egg substitute or 2 tablespoons of apple sauce.

7. To make all gluten free, use your favorite 1:1 gluten free all purpose flour or oat flour.

2. Crustless Blueberry Pie

Prep Time: 15 Minutes

Cook Time: 50 Minutes

Servings: 8

Ingredients

- 1 cup all purpose flour
- ½ cup white sugar
- ¼ cup brown sugar
- ½ teaspoon ground cinnamon
- pinch of nutmeg
- ¼ teaspoon salt
- ½ cup unsalted butter, melted
- 2 large eggs
- 1.5 teaspoons vanilla extract
- 2 ¼ cups frozen blueberries
- 1 tablespoon brown sugar for topping

Instructions

1. Preheat oven to 350F. Use a butter wrapper to grease the inside of a 9-inch round pie dish. Set aside

2. In a large bowl, add flour, sugars, cinnamon, nutmeg, and salt, and whisk to combine. In a medium bowl add the melted butter (melt in the microwave about 30 seconds). Wait for the butter to cool before mixing in the eggs to avoid cooking them. Add the eggs, vanilla extract, and whisk with a fork.

3. Pour the wet mixture into the dry and stir to combine. Add frozen blueberries, stirring till blueberries are mixed through evenly. The dough might get a bit difficult to stir, but just keep stirring and it will loosen.

4. Pour batter into the greased pie dish. Sprinkle 1 tablespoon sugar over the top. Bake for about 50 to 60 minutes, or until edges are slightly brown and a toothpick inserted in the center comes out clean or with a few moist crumbs but no batter.

5. Allow pie to cool before slicing and serving. Serve with whipped cream or vanilla ice cream.

6. Gluten free all purpose flour can be substituted in this recipe, however, I find this sometimes increases the baking time needed.

7. You can also use fresh blueberries - I have used 2 cups fresh and ¼ cup frozen. You can also mix regular blueberries and wild blueberries for a more tart flavor.

8. Store at room temperature for 1 day and then transfer to the fridge or freezer.

3. Homemade Cereal Bars

Prep Time: 5 Minutes

Cook Time: 5 Minutes

Servings: 12

Ingredients

- 3 cups cereal of your choice like rice or corn chex, cheerios, etc. slightly crushed (I used 2 cups of chex and 1 cup of cheerios)
- ¼ cup honey
- ¼ cup maple syrup
- ½ cup sunflower seed butter
- 1 cup white chocolate

Optional:

- Pinch of salt and 1 teaspoon of cinnamon sprinkled on top

Instructions

1. Line an 8x8 inch pan with parchment paper (up the sides). In a medium pot, add honey and maple syrup. Bring to a low simmer (small bubbles) over medium heat for 1-2 minutes. Lower heat and add sunflower seed butter until combined and creamy. Add a pinch of salt if your sunbutter isn't salted. Off the heat, add your cereal and stir to fully coat.

2. Spoon the cereal mixture into your 8x8 inch pan and press down slightly to set everything together. Place your white chocolate in a bowl and microwave in 30 second intervals, stirring after each interval until fully melted. Spread the white chocolate evenly on top. If you'd like, sprinkle 1 teaspoon of cinnamon on top of the white chocolate.

3. Refrigerate up to 2 hours or overnight for best results. To cut, lift the bars from the square pan by holding the parchment paper. With a large knife, slice large sections, then go back to slice smaller squares. Store and serve chilled.

4. For gluten free, choose certified gluten free cereals.

5. For dairy free, use Enjoy Life white chocolate.

6. This makes a very thin white chocolate crust. For a thicker coating, melt more white chocolate (1 ½-2 cups).

7. Be sure to not overcook the white chocolate in the microwave, which will cause the chocolate to "seize up". Stopping often to stir frequently until JUST melted will produce smooth results.

8. If bars do not stay together the honey/maple mixture was not simmered long enough or they need more time to cool.

4. Easy Quiche Florentine

Prep Time: 15 Minutes

Cook Time: 50 Minutes

Servings: 4

Ingredients

- 1 9" frozen pie crust
- 3 large eggs
- ¾ cup whole milk
- ¼ cup heavy cream
- 3 oz chevre (soft goat cheese)
- ½ cup loosely chopped fresh spinach
- 1 shallot, chopped
- ¼-1/2 teaspoon kosher salt and black pepper
- fresh thyme (optional)

Instructions

1. Remove pie crust from freezer and allow it to warm while you preheat your oven. When softened a bit, poke holes all around the crust with the tines of a

fork. If you want your crust to not puff up even more, fill it with pie weights or beans. Pre-bake your pie crust according to package directions (mine was 425 degrees F for 15-20 minutes) on the bottom ⅓rd of your oven, until very lightly browned.

2. Meanwhile, mix together the eggs, milk, cream and whisk till combined. Then add goat cheese (crumble with your fingers), spinach, and chopped shallot with kosher salt and black pepper and stir. The goat cheese will not fully combine, but that's ok, it will melt down.

3. Remove pre-baked pie crust from the oven, change the temperature to 400 degrees F, and pour in the filling. It's really ok if you pie bottom breaks a part a bit, you won't be able to tell once it's baked.

4. Bake at 400 degrees F for about 50 minutes, until the center is puffed up. It should have just a slight jiggle, not a wave, when you move it around. Allow it to set/cool for about 5-10 minutes before eating. I LOVE a little fresh thyme leaves on top if you have them on hand.

5. Pre-baking your frozen pie crust is necessary to keep it from having a soggy bottom. I also find that baking in the lower ⅓rd of my oven helps as well.

6. I have never had an issue with my crust burning at these cooking times, but if yours is looking a little dark, you can cover the crust with tin foil or a crust shield, if you have it.

7. Gluten free pie crusts are fairly easy to locate. I would not recommend editing this recipe to be dairy-free.

8. For those sensitive to histamine, replace the spinach with chopped lacinato kale.

5. Banana Applesauce Muffins

Prep Time: 10 Minutes

Cook Time: 35 Minutes

Servings: 11

Ingredients

- 3 medium bananas (speckled or brown)
- 3 tablespoons extra virgin olive oil
- 2 tablespoons melted butter
- ⅓ cup unsweetened applesauce
- 1 teaspoon vanilla
- 2 tablespoons sugar
- 1 teaspoon cinnamon
- ½ teaspoon nutmeg
- 1 large egg
- 1½ cups all purpose flour or gluten free 1:1 baking flour
- 1 teaspoon baking soda
- 1 teaspoon baking powder
- ¼ teaspoon salt

- Rolled oats for garnish, if desired.

Instructions

1. Start by preheating the oven to 350 degrees Fahrenheit (180 C). In a large bowl, begin by mashing the peeled bananas with a fork. Some small chunks can remain, but try to mash it enough for an even texture. Stir in melted butter, olive oil, applesauce, spices, sugar, and vanilla until fully combined. Then mix in one egg.

2. On top of the wet ingredients, add flour, baking powder, salt, and baking soda. Then gently stir that into the wet ingredients. A dough mixer can make this very easy!

3. Fill a muffin tin with liners and spoon the muffin mixture into each, filling about ¾ full. This should create 11-12 muffins. Sprinkle a small pinch of oats on top, if desired.

4. Bake for 15-17 minutes, till just light brown on top and set. The muffins may appear a little underdone, but will continue cooking after you remove them from the oven. This will retain a moist texture.

Allow the muffins to cool at least 5 minutes before removing them from the pan and serving.

5. For an accurate flour measurement, scoop the flour into a measuring cup with a spoon, then level with a knife. Do not directly scoop the measuring cup into the flour.

6. Because of the low sugar added to this recipe, make sure the bananas have browned at least enough to be speckled and are not a green color.

7. This is part of my reintroduction series, and bananas are not a part of the elimination period. To replace, use 1 cup pumpkin puree or try my Cinnamon Oatmeal Muffins.

6. Beef Protein Bowl

Prep Time: 10 Minutes

Cook Time: 25 Minutes

Servings: 3

Ingredients

- 1 pound ground beef
- salt and black pepper
- olive oil
- 8 oz cauliflower rice
- ½ teaspoon chili powder
- ½ teaspoon cumin
- ½ teaspoon smoked paprika
- 2 zucchini squash, cut into cubes
- 1 cup spinach
- 2 large eggs
- 2 green onion, chopped
- salsa verde or any salsa

Instructions

1. In a large non stick pan, cook ground beef over medium high heat, stirring frequently, till cooked through and crumbly - about 5-6 minutes total. Season with a pinch of salt and pepper, then remove from the pan and set aside.

2. In the same pan, add a teaspoon of olive oil and cauliflower rice, along with the chili powder, cumin, and smoked paprika. Cook for 1-2 minutes over medium heat, then add the zucchini, cooking another 2-3 minutes till just barely softened. Add ¼ teaspoon of kosher salt and a pinch of fresh pepper and set aside.

3. Carefully wipe out the pan with a paper towel and add another teaspoon of olive oil over medium high heat. Crack the eggs and carefully lay them into the pan so the yolk doesn't break apart. Allow the egg to cook till the whites are set, then flip and cook another 20-40 seconds for an over easy/medium egg. Meanwhile, use the other side of pan to wilt the spinach just slightly.

4. In a bowl, add the cauliflower rice and zucchini, top with the ground beef, then add the eggs and spinach. Taste and adjust any seasonings and then

add your favorite salsa and top with chopped green onions.

5. This is my favorite salsa verde, but I really like Tacodeli's Salsa Verde for a store-bought option.

6. I used Trader fresh cauliflower rice for this recipe and used ½ a bag, approximately 8oz.

7. For extra flavor, also season your beef using this ground beef taco seasoning recipe.

8. If you're not following a migraine diet or have reintroduced foods, sliced avocado is a wonderful addition, as well as a little bit of lime juice on top.

7. Pumpkin Apple Bread

Prep Time: 15 Minutes

Cook Time: 1 hrs 5 Minutes

Servings: 8

Ingredients

- 2 cups all purpose flour
- 1 teaspoon baking soda
- 2 teaspoons cinnamon
- 2 teaspoons pumpkin spice
- 1 teaspoon table salt
- 2 large eggs
- ¾ cup white sugar
- ½ cup light brown sugar
- 1 15oz can pumpkin puree (not pie filling)
- ½ cup vegetable or canola oil
- ¼ cup apple juice
- ⅔ cup honeycrisp apples (about 1 apple), chopped small

Instructions

1. Adjust your oven rack to the lower ⅓rd of your oven. Preheat to 350°F degrees. Grease a 9x5 loaf pan well with extra oil. In one large bowl, combine the flour, baking soda, cinnamon, pumpkin spice, and salt and mix till combined.

2. In a small bowl, whisk the eggs and add white and brown sugar, mixing till combined. In another separate bowl, combine the pumpkin puree with oil and apple juice till smooth. Fold in the egg/sugar mixture, then mix the wet ingredients into the dry ingredients. There will be a few lumps, this is ok. Finally add in the apples, stirring till just combined.

3. Pour the batter into the prepared loaf pan and bake uncovered for 30 minutes on the lower rack. Add a tented tin foil cover, so it gives the bread enough room to rise more. Bake another 30-35 minutes until a toothpick inserted in the center comes out almost clean. Allow it to cool 10-15 minutes before removing from the baking pan. It should slide right out if oiled correctly, but running a knife along the sides to loosen it may help.

4. I love honeycrisp apples in this recipe. I used honeycrisp apple juice from North Coast and 1 apple, however, other types of apples/apple juice will work fine for this recipe. Something a little sweet is best.

5. If following a migraine diet, check your pumpkin spice label for lemon. I used Simply Organics.

6. This recipe freezes very well. I let thaw at room temperature or microwave for 10-15 seconds.

8. Thai Noodle Salad with Sunflower "Peanut" Dressing

Prep Time: 25 Minutes

Cook Time: 30 Minutes

Servings: 4

Ingredients

For the salad:

- 8 oz pad thai rice noodles
- 1 ½ cups cabbage slaw mix
- 1 red bell pepper, cut into thin strips
- 2 green onions, chopped
- ¼ cup cilantro, chopped
- ¼ cup basil, chopped
- ½ watermelon radish, or 2-3 small red radish, cut into strips

For the sunflower seed dressing:

- ¼ cup sunflower seed butter

- ¼ cup unsweetened pomegranate or tart cherry juice
- 2-3 tablespoons distilled white vinegar
- 2 tablespoons coconut aminos
- 2 tablespoons sesame oil
- 2 tablespoons honey
- 2 teaspoons fresh grated ginger
- 1 minced garlic clove
- salt and pepper to taste
- sriracha or sweet chili sauce to taste (optional)

Instructions

1. Cook the rice noodles according to package directions, drain, and run under cool water to cool down. If the noodles are sticking together, add a tiny bit of sesame oil and toss them in it.
2. While you're waiting for the noodles to cook, add the sunflower seed butter, juice, vinegar, coconut aminos, sesame oil, honey, ginger, and garlic to a food processor. Blend until totally smooth and creamy. Taste and add kosher salt and pepper, as needed. (This will vary as some sunflower seed butters are more salty or sweet than others). Set

aside to let the flavors meld together, about 30 minutes.

3. Place the cooled noodles in a large bowl with slaw, chopped bell pepper, cilantro, basil, and radish. Chill everything for 30 minutes while you wait for the dressing to develop some flavor. Then add the dressing a little bit at a time, tossing everything together until it's dressed to your liking (you may have some leftover). Serve cold with sriracha and/or sweet chili sauce on the side.

4. This salad will keep in the fridge for 2 days.

9. Boursin Broccoli Rice Casserole

Prep Time: 30 Minutes

Cook Time: 20 Minutes

Servings: 6

Ingredients

- 2 cups pre-cooked brown rice I added this 30 min into your prep time. Follow your rice package directions.
- 1 tablespoon unsalted butter or olive oil
- 2 medium shallots, peeled and chopped
- 1 garlic clove, peeled and minced
- 2 tablespoons all purpose flour
- 1 cup whole milk
- ½ cup vegetable or chicken stock
- 12 oz fresh broccoli florets
- 1 5oz Boursin garlic and herb cheese package
- ½ cup panko
- salt and fresh pepper to taste

Instructions

1. Preheat oven to 400 degrees. In a large pot, bring water to a boil. Add broccoli florets and cook for 1 minute. Remove broccoli immediately (drain hot water), and run under cold water. Pat dry.

2. In a large saucepan, melt a tablespoon of butter or olive oil over medium heat. Add shallots and garlic and cook for about a minute. Then add flour and stir to combine. Slowly add in your broth, whisking as you add it. Then add in your milk a little bit at a time, whisking after each addition to make sure it smooths out. Remove the pan from heat and whisk in your Boursin cheese block. Taste the sauce to make sure you like the seasonings and add a little kosher salt and pepper.

3. Stir in the broccoli florets and rice. Place mixture into an 8x8 casserole dish (or something similar). Top with panko. Cook for about 15-20 minutes, until panko is lightly browned on top.

4. To make this recipe gluten free, use rice flour instead of the all purpose and substitute gluten free panko.

10. Dairy Free Quiche with Leeks and Sausage

Prep Time: 15 Minutes

Cook Time: 30 Minutes

Servings: 12

Ingredients

- ⅓ cup leeks, washed and chopped
- ¾ cup cooked sausage
- 4 large eggs
- ½ cup oat milk
- ¼ teaspoon dried thyme leaves
- ½ teaspoon kosher salt and black pepper to taste (about ¼ tsp)
- 1 pre-made 9" pie dough (flat, not in a large pie form) at room temperature
- oil for greasing the muffin tin

Instructions

1. Preheat oven to 375 degrees F. Begin by washing your chopped leeks well, draining and drying. In a medium bowl, combine the leeks, cooked sausage, eggs, oat milk, thyme, salt, and pepper, whisking till well combined.

2. Meanwhile form the pie dough and roll it out with a rolling pin to about 1/8-1/4" thickness. Use a 3 inch glass or cookie cutter to cut circles in the dough and put into a greased or non-stick muffin tin. You will probably have to do this in two steps, rolling out the remaining pie dough again to use the rest. Press along the sides of a greased muffin tin so the dough is thin (it does not need to reach the top). You should have enough for all 12 tins.

3. Pour the egg filling into the quiche dough, evenly dispersing among the cups, and bake for 25-30 minutes until cooked through and set on top. Allow to cool in the muffin tin for 5 minutes and then slide a knife around the edges, carefully lifting the quiche out the pan. Serve warm and enjoy!

4. I recommend using a dark nonstick muffin tin. If you don't, it may require longer cooking time or pre-baking the crust.

5. For this recipe I like to use my sausage recipe (pg53 of my cookbook) or pre-made fresh sweet Italian chicken sausage from whole foods, sprouts, Central Market or trader joe's. These would be the kind that are uncooked with fresh ground meat, usually sold behind the meat counter, and not the kind in sealed packages that have the texture of hot dogs. This makes this recipe migraine diet compliant.

6. Make sure your dough is at room temperature or it won't be easy to work with.

11. Ahi Tuna Salad with Sesame Dressing

Prep Time: 30 Minutes

Cook Time: 20 Minutes

Servings: 4

Ingredients

Sesame Crusted Ahi Tuna:

- 2 ahi tuna steaks
- 3 tablespoons mild cooking oil (I use sesame or grapeseed)
- 2 tablespoons coconut aminos
- 1 teaspoon rice flour
- ¼ cup organic pear juice
- 2 tablespoons honey
- 1 teaspoon sriracha hot sauce
- ⅓ cup white and/or black sesame seeds, toasted

Salad:

- 4-5 oz mixed greens

- 1 large mango, sliced
- 1 large radish, sliced
- ⅓ cup green onions, chopped (about 1-2)
- Sesame Ginger Dressing
- ¼ cup toasted sesame oil
- 1 tablespoons coconut aminos
- 2 tablespoons pear juice
- 1 tablespoon white vinegar
- 1½ tablespoons tahini
- 1-2 teaspoons ginger (if using fresh use 2 teaspoons and if using dried use 1 teaspoon)
- 1 clove garlic, minced
- salt and pepper to taste I used about 1 tsp

Instructions

1. For the dressing, whisk all ingredients together till very smooth, or for best results put them in a small food processor and blend. Allow to sit in the fridge for at least 30 minutes for the flavors to combine. If sesame seeds aren't toasted

2. For the ahi tuna sauce, combine the coconut aminos, flour, pear juice, honey, and sriracha in a small pot. Heat over medium high heat until simmering. Allow to simmer till thickened, about 5 minutes.

3. In another non-stick or cast iron pan, heat oil over medium-high heat. Lightly salt both sides of the ahi and add to the pan. Sear for 1-2 minutes on the first side, flip and brush with the thickened sauce. Sear another 1-2 minutes for rare to medium rare. For medium, sear 3 minutes. Remove the ahi steak the pan and brush the just cooked side with the remaining sauce.

4. Spread your sesame seeds on a plate and lay your tuna on them, coating both sides of the fish. Slice very thin.

5. Combine the lettuce and a spoonful of the dressing, tossing till well-coated. Place the seared tuna on top with the radish, green onion, and mango.

6. If you can't find pear juice, apple juice will work in a pinch. But I would highly recommend trying for the best flavor.

7. Toast the sesame seeds by either broiling on high heat and watching VERY carefully for about 1-2 minutes or heating them in a dry skillet over medium heat till very lightly browned.

8. Purchase frozen sushi grade or good quality fresh ahi tuna from a trusted fishmonger. Remember raw or undercooked fish does increase the risk of foodborne illness, so purchasing good quality is essential.

9. The longer the fish sits after cooking, the more it will cook through on the inside. If you want this just barely seared, cook for 1 minute on both sides and slice quickly. If you'd like your tuna more cooked through, cook 2 minutes on the first side and 2-3 on the second.

10. If not following a migraine diet, you can substitute soy sauce for coconut aminos, however, the recipe will be much more sodium heavy. I would

recommend balancing it with some sweetness like extra honey.

12. Halloumi Couscous Salad

Prep Time: 15 Minutes

Cook Time: 24 Minutes

Servings: 6

Ingredients

Halloumi Couscous Salad

- 1 cup couscous
- 2 fresh corn cobs, kernels removed
- 1 cup seedless cucumber, chopped
- 2 green onion, chopped
- ½ 15oz can low sodium black beans
- ¾ cup chopped tomatoes
- 1½ cups arugula or spinach (or just a large handful)
- 8 oz halloumi cheese

Creamy Dijon Dressing:

- 1 tablespoon shallot, minced
- ⅓ cup extra virgin olive oil
- 2 tablespoons vinegar

- 1 tablespoon apple juice
- 2 teaspoons dijon mustard
- 1 teaspoon mayonnaise
- 2 teaspoons honey
- salt and black pepper to taste

Instructions

1. In a large, shallow pan with a lid, add 1 cup of water and bring to a simmer over medium heat. Stir in couscous and corn kernels, cover, and turn off the heat. Let it sit for 10 minutes, then remove lid and fluff with a spoon.

2. Meanwhile place all the ingredients for the dressing in a small mason jar and shake till creamy and well-mixed (or whisk). Add the cucumber, green onions, black beans, tomatoes, and arugula to a large bowl, along with the couscous.

3. Carefully use a paper towel soaked with vegetable or avocado oil to rub the grill grates and preheat the grill to medium high heat. Add halloumi cheese, sliced in half if very thick, and grill for 4-5 minutes per side or until grill marks form and the cheese begins to soften inside.

4. Toss couscous and vegetables with a little bit of the dressing (taste and see how much you like before adding in the entire dressing). Season with salt and freshly cracked black pepper to taste, but go easy on the salt because halloumi will fill in what you're missing. Serve with the halloumi in whole pieces or sliced.

5. Quinoa can be substituted for couscous for a gluten free option.

6. For extra flavor, I love to simmer vegetable broth instead of water which helps flavor the couscous even more.

7. Trader Joe's has the best price on halloumi that I have seen.

8. For a low sodium alternative, use mozzarella balls instead of halloumi (but don't grill them).

9. Wait to toss the dressing till the end so the vegetables don't get soggy.

10. For migraine-friendly, use a sulfite-free dijon mustard.

13. Tuna Pesto Pasta

Prep Time: 5 Minutes

Cook Time: 30 Minutes

Servings: 5

Ingredients

- 10-12 oz pasta (linguine, fusilli, spaghetti, or penne recommended)
- 6.7oz canned or bottled tuna
- ¾ cup pesto (homemade or store-bought)
- ¼ cup leftover pasta water

Homemade Pesto:

- ⅓ cup rosted pepitas or sunflower seeds
- 1 clove garlic
- 2 cups spinach and arugula blend
- 1 cup fresh basil leaves
- ⅓ cup extra virgin olive oil
- 2 teaspoons white vinegar
- ¼ teaspoon kosher salt and black pepper to taste

Instructions

1. If using homemade pesto, all all ingredients to a food processor and blend till combined, seed particles should be even and small. Meanwhile bring a large pot of salted water to a boil and add pasta. Cook according to package directions, then drain, reserving about ¼ to ½ cup of the pasta water.

2. In a large bowl, combine pesto and tuna. Stir in warm pasta, and ¼ cup of the pasta water, till everything is fully coated with the tuna and pesto sauce. Taste and adjust any seasonings. Serve warm or cover and refrigerate to serve as a pasta salad.

3. For a more "saucy" pasta, add more pasta water as desired, about 1 tablespoon at a time.

4. Basil turns black with a lot of heat. It should be fine with the pasta and a little bit of water, but be mindful when reheating. Especially in the microwave. This is also why we toss the pesto in a bowl rather than on the stove.

5. To preserve the flavor and color, I recommend serving leftovers cold or at room temperature.

6. A squeeze of lemon is delicious, if tolerated!

14. Spicy Salmon Bowl

Prep Time: 25 Minutes

Cook Time: 10 Minutes

Servings: 4

Ingredients

Marinated Salmon:

- 1½ pounds fresh salmon, skin off, cut into 1 inch cubes
- ⅓ cup coconut aminos
- 1 tablespoon toasted sesame oil
- 1 garlic clove, minced

Bowls:

- 2 tablespoons distilled white vinegar
- 1 tablespoon coconut aminos
- 8 oz bag shredded cabbage/slaw mix
- 20 oz bag microwavable rice, brown or white
- 1 cup shredded carrots
- ½ english (seedless) cucumber, sliced

- 2 tablespoons toasted sesame seeds and/or panko

Spicy Mayo:

- ⅓ cup mayonnaise

- 1 tablespoon sriracha

- 1 teaspoon distilled white vinegar or lime juice

Instructions

1. In a medium bowl, combine salmon, coconut aminos, toasted sesame oil, and garlic. Stir to combine and place in the fridge for at least 30 minutes to marinate.

2. Meanwhile, stir together the mayonnaise, sriracha, and vinegar - adjusting to your taste for spice level. Set aside. Stir together the coconut aminos and vinegar, then toss the cabbage with the mixture, thoroughly coating the cabbage, and set in the refrigerator till ready to use. Microwave the rice and chop the vegetables.

3. Over medium heat, add salmon to a large non-stick or carbon steel pan, leaving space between pieces to sear. Adjusting heat to medium-medium high to sear on first side for about 2 minutes till a nice

caramelization forms on the outside. Don't mess with the salmon or move it around, or it may stick and not sear properly.

4. Using tongs, flip salmon to the other side and cook another 2 minutes till cooked through to a medium temperature (or cook longer if you want it to be cooked through). You may need to work in batches, so set a plate with a paper towel next to the pan and remove the salmon pieces as they're finished.

5. Build your bowl - Add rice and slaw to the bottom, then top with carrots, cucumber, and salmon. Drizzle with spicy mayo and top with panko and/or sesame seeds.

6. If you are sensitive to coconut aminos, leave them out of the recipe. It won't have the same sweetness, but will still be good.

7. To make this salmon bowl low carb, use cauliflower rice or double the amount of cabbage and use that as a base.

8. The oil from the salmon marinade should be enough to sear it in, however, if you have a pan that isn't nonstick, oil the pan accordingly.

15. Blackened Cod

Prep Time: 5 Minutes

Cook Time: 10 Minutes

Servings: 4

Ingredients

Blackened Cod:

- 2 teaspoons chili powder
- 1 teaspoon garlic powder
- ½ teaspoon oregano
- 1 teaspoon paprika
- 1 teaspoon kosher salt (or less, if low sodium)
- ¼ teaspoon cayenne*
- 1 ½ pounds fresh cod filet, skin removed
- mild oil or butter for frying

Coleslaw:

- ⅓ cup mayonnaise
- 1 tablespoon distilled white vinegar
- 1 teaspoon honey

- ¼ teaspoon cumin
- 8 oz shredded cabbage mix
- 1 green onion, chopped
- ¼ cup shredded carrots
- salt and pepper to taste

Instructions

1. In a small bowl, mix together the chili powder, garlic powder, oregano, paprika, kosher salt, and cayenne (if using). Cut cod into 4 servings of filets and pat both sides with the spice mixture.

2. Using a cast iron pan, heat 1-2 tablespoons of butter or oil over medium high heat. When oil is shimmering and hot, add the seasoned cod and sear for 5 minutes, until blackened and crispy. Flip and cook another 4-5 minutes until blackened and cooked through.

3. Meanwhile combine the mayonnaise, vinegar, honey and cumin and whisk till smooth. Toss with the cabbage, green onion, and carrots. Place in the fridge for at least 5 minutes to allow flavors to combine and cabbage to soften. Serve coleslaw under the fish.

4. If you don't like your fish spicy, simply omit the cayenne. It will still have some heat from the chili powder, but not be too spicy.

5. For low sodium, you can edit the amount of salt used.

6. If you don't own a cast iron pan, it's ok. You may just not get as great of a dark crust on the fish. However, it will be important to preheat your pan to high heat.

16. Grilled Italian Shrimp

Prep Time: 10 Minutes

Cook Time: 35 Minutes

Servings: 3

Ingredients

- 2 large garlic cloves, peeled
- 2 tablespoons fresh basil
- 1 tablespoon fresh parsley
- 1.5 teaspoon dried thyme
- 1 teaspoon honey
- 1 tablespoon tomato paste
- 3 tablespoons extra virgin olive oil
- 1.5 tablespoons distilled white vinegar
- ½ teaspoon salt
- 1 pound peeled and deveined jumbo or extra large RAW shrimp, tail on * fresh or frozen and defrosted is fine
- fresh black pepper to taste

Instructions

1. If your shrimp does not come deveined, this is pretty easy to do. Remove the shell (which is usually already cut) and use a small knife to cut along the back side of the shrimp. There will be a slimy dark "line" that becomes exposed. Remove that from the shrimp and rinse. Pat the shrimp dry.

2. Place all the ingredients except shrimp in a food processor and blend it till almost smooth. Pour sauce over the shrimp, toss, and place in the refrigerator to marinate 30min to an hour. If using a grill, thread your shrimp onto skewers.

3. Prepare your grill or grill pan to medium high heat. Place your shrimp on the hot grill or grill pan and cook, not moving for 2 minutes. Flip and cook on the other side another 2-3 minutes, depending on the size of your shrimp. You want them to be opaque with no clear/grayish parts. Serve immediately or cover and chill for up to 2 days.

4. sIf you're sensitive to tomatoes, simply remove the tomato paste from the marinade. It's not quite as good, but still really flavorful and delicious.

5. Make sure the shrimp is completely defrosted before using. You can defrost quickly in a bowl of

cold water, changing the water out every 20 minutes until shrimp have defrosted.

6. I love to pair this with a pasta salad, mozzarella salad, or mashed cauliflower.

17. Crockpot BBQ Chicken Thighs

Prep Time: 5 Minutes

Cook Time: 2 hrs 5 Minutes

Servings: 4

Ingredients

- 2 large shallots, chopped
- 2 garlic cloves, minced
- 2 tablespoons apple juice
- 1½ cups strained tomatoes
- 1½ tablespoons brown sugar
- 1 tablespoon smoked paprika
- ½ teaspoon dry mustard
- ⅛ teaspoon cayenne pepper
- kosher salt and pepper to taste (I typically start with adding 1 teaspoon to the slow cooker before cooking)
- 2 pounds boneless, skinless chicken thighs

Instructions

1. Start by adding your chopped shallots and garlic to the slow cooker, along with the apple juice, strained tomatoes, brown sugar, smoked paprika, dry mustard, and cayenne pepper (if using). Lay the chicken thighs on top, then turn them to coat with the sauce.

2. Place the lid on the slow cooker and cook on low for 2-3 hours till cooked through (an internal temperature of 165°F). Remove the chicken thighs and serve whole, or shred with two forks for a shredded BBQ sandwich. Taste and adjust any seasonings.

3. I like Pomi brand of strained tomatoes. Look for one without seasonings.

4. Temperatures on slow cookers can vary greatly. If yours cooks fast, err on the low end of cooking time (like mine does).

5. You can use bone in chicken thighs, they will just add another hour to the cooking time.

6. In a pinch, you can use high heat and cut the time in half, however, the meal won't be quite as flavorful, and might be a little more dry. Same notes go for using chicken breasts.

18. Green Enchilada Chicken Soup

Prep Time: 20 Minutes

Cook Time: 15 Minutes

Servings: 4

Ingredients

- 1 pound tomatillos
- 3-4 garlic cloves
- 1 poblano, de-seeded and sliced in half
- ⅔ cup chopped shallots
- 4 cups vegetable or chicken broth
- 2 teaspoons cumin
- 2 teaspoons oregano
- 1 teaspoon coriander
- 1 teaspoon kosher salt
- ¾ pound cooked, shredded chicken *I use a "naked" rotisserie chicken, meaning no spices added
- ½ cup fresh cilantro, chopped
- fresh tortillas or tortilla chips

Instructions

1. Preheat broiler to high heat. Remove paper skins and stems from tomatillos and wash under warm water to remove sticky residue. You can leave the garlic skin on for broiling. Place the tomatillos, garlic, and poblano on a baking sheet and broil about 6-10 inches away from heat for 6 minutes. Flip tomatillos and remove the poblano and garlic if softened and charred in spots. Peel skin off garlic. Continue broiling the tomatillos until softened and charred in spots, another 6 minutes.

2. Meanwhile prep a large soup pot. Add the charred tomatillos, garlic, and poblano to the pot along with the chopped shallots and saute over medium heat about 2 minutes until the shallots have softened. Add 4 cups of broth, cumin, oregano, coriander, and salt. Stir to combine and bring to a boil, then decrease the heat to simmer for 10 minutes. Add chopped cilantro. With an immersion blender, blend the soup in the pot till it reaches your desired consistency (I like mine smooth). Stir in chicken and adjust any seasonings to your liking.

3. To serve, top with crispy tortilla chips, or toast fresh tortillas brushed on both sides with a little bit

of olive oil at 400 degrees F for about 7-10 minutes until light brown. They'll crisp up as they cool.

4. Canned tomatillos can be substituted for fresh, but fresh are preferable.

5. See notes in post for gluten free/vegetarian/vegan.

6. You can find naked chickens at Sprouts, Whole Foods, and Fresh Market but any plain, cooked chicken will do.

19. Boursin Broccoli Soup

Prep Time: 15 Minutes

Cook Time: 25 Minutes

Servings: 4

Ingredients

- ¼ cup butter
- 2 large shallots, chopped
- 2 large carrots, chopped small (1 cup)
- ¼ cup all purpose flour (gluten free if needed)
- 3 cups vegetable broth
- 1 ½ cups whole milk*
- 1 head broccoli chopped into florets (about 2 full cups florets)
- 5 oz Boursin Garlic & Herb cheese
- ¾ teaspoon kosher salt (or omit for lower sodium)
- ½ teaspoon black pepper

Instructions

1. In a large, heavy pot (I used a 5 ½ quart pot), melt the butter over medium heat and stir in chopped shallots and carrots. Saute for about 2 minutes until they are fragrant and more tender, stirring often. Add ¼ cup of flour and coat the vegetables. Pour in about ½ cup of broth and whisk till the flour gets incorporated and smooth. Then add the rest of the broth as well as the whole milk. Bring to a low simmer for 8-10 minutes, allowing it to thicken. Do not start to boil, otherwise your milk might curdle (especially if using a low fat option instead).

2. Add the broccoli florets and cook for another 5 minutes until softened. Off the heat, stir in Boursin cheese until smooth and creamy. Taste and adjust any seasonings, like salt and pepper if needed.

3. I recommend using whole milk to give the soup extra creaminess and also the higher fat content makes it less likely to curdle, however you can use any milk substitute you'd like. Just be aware!

20. Healthy Sloppy (without Ketchup)

Prep Time: 10 Minutes

Cook Time: 25 Minutes

Servings: 4

Ingredients

- 1 pound ground beef
- 3 garlic cloves, minced
- 1 large shallot, chopped
- ½ cup chopped poblano pepper
- ½ teaspoon kosher salt
- 1 ⅓ cups strained tomatoes (plain tomato puree)
- 2 tablespoons coconut aminos
- 1 tablespoon mustard (dijon also works)
- 1 tablespoon distilled white vinegar
- ½ teaspoon smoked paprika
- 4 Burger buns (or baked potatoes)

Instructions

1. In a large saute pan, cook ground beef over medium heat until cooked through, about 5-6 minutes. Drain any excess liquid/fat. Add minced garlic, shallots, and chopped poblano, cooking another 5 minutes until pepper has softened. Stir often so the garlic doesn't burn. Add salt, if desired, and strained tomatoes, coconut aminos, mustard, vinegar, and paprika along with ⅓ cup of water.

2. Bring to a simmer and allow it to simmer for 10 minutes, until the sauce has thickened. If it starts getting too thick, just add a little more water.

3. If you're sensitive to spicy food, consider cutting back on the amount of poblano pepper. Some are more spicy than others, but overall this pepper is very mild so ½ cup should yield a very light heat without burning your mouth.

4. If sensitive to sodium, adjust the amount of salt and check your coconut aminos for one that's lower.

5. I used Pomi brand strained tomatoes. These are just pureed tomatoes, like a thick tomato sauce with nothing added.

6. This recipe is great doubled or tripled for meal prep and freezes well.

21. Beef Stew without Wine

Prep Time: 10 Minutes

Cook Time: 1 hrs 30 Minutes

Servings: 6

Ingredients

- 2.75 pounds boneless beef chuck roast cut into bite sized pieces
- splash of olive oil
- 2 tablespoons butter or olive oil
- 2 large shallots, chopped
- 2 celery stalks, chopped
- 3 carrots, peeled and chopped
- 3 garlic cloves, minced
- 3 yukon gold potatoes, cut into 1" pieces
- 2 tablespoons flour
- 2 sprigs fresh rosemary
- ½ teaspoon dried thyme
- 2 bay leaves

- 5 cups low sodium beef or vegetable broth
- kosher salt and pepper

Instructions

1. In a large dutch oven, splash a bit of olive oil and turn to medium high heat. Season beef with kosher salt and black pepper. Add chopped beef chuck roast in batches, leaving enough space so it browns and doesn't steam. Brown on all sides, about 5-6 minutes total. Repeat with any leftover meat.

2. Remove the meat and leave the drippings. Add 2 tablespoons butter or olive oil to the dutch oven along with shallots, celery, and carrots. Stir occasionally over medium heat until softened, about 3 minutes. Add garlic and mix into the vegetables. Then add the potatoes and beef. Stir in flour with a wood spoon until fully mixed in, coating all the beef and vegetables.

3. Stir in rosemary, thyme, bay leaves, ½ teaspoon kosher salt, and finally all the broth (or any other liquid additions you're using). Bring everything to a boil over high heat and reduce heat to low. Cover and cook on low heat (or enough for a low simmer)

for about 1.5 hours or until the beef is tender and flavors have combined. Taste and adjust any seasonings. Remove bay leaves and rosemary stalks before serving.

4. For beef broth, I recommend Butcher's Bone Broth. For vegetable broth I recommend Trader Joe's Hearty Vegetable or the recipe from my cookbook.

5. If using vegetable broth, I recommend adding ¼ cup of coconut aminos when adding the broth for a greater depth of flavor. Tart cherry juice can also be used as a "red wine" replacement. See post for more details.

6. For gluten free, use all purpose GF flour or cornstarch.

7. This can also be made in the oven (in a covered dutch oven) at 325 degrees F for roughly 2 hours.

22. Stir Fry Without Soy Sauce

Prep Time: 15 Minutes

Cook Time: 12 Minutes

Servings: 4

Ingredients

Soy Free Sesame Sauce:

- ½ cup coconut aminos
- 3 tablespoons tahini
- 1 teaspoon distilled white vinegar
- 1 teaspoon toasted sesame oil
- 2 cloves garlic, minced
- 1½-2 teaspoons ground mustard The more you use, the more spicy the dish will be.
- 1 teaspoon peeled and grated fresh ginger
- salt to taste

Stir Fry:

- Vegetable oil spray
- 2 lbs boneless, skinless chicken breast or thighs, cut into bite-size pieces

- 1 cup zucchini, washed and chopped into ½" pieces
- ¾ cup carrots, chopped
- ⅓ cup red pepper, chopped
- ½ cup broccoli florets
- 4 oz mushrooms (optional)

Instructions

1. Add all the sauce ingredients to a food processor and blend till combined, or mix with a whisk till smooth. Taste and see if you need to add salt. Salt will balance the sweetness of the coconut aminos. Set aside.

2. Spray a large skillet or wok with oil and set to medium high heat. Add chicken and sear on first side for about 3 minutes, getting a nice caramelization. Use a wood spoon to flip and cook another 3-4 minutes, or until cooked through. Transfer cooked chicken to a plate.

3. Spray oil again to the same skillet or wok. If there are brown bits of chicken att the bottom, use a splash or broth or sauce to lift them up from the bottom of the pan. Add all the vegges except for the mushrooms and cook on medium high heat for 3-4

minutes. Move them to the side of the pan and add the mushrooms, cooking another 2 minutes.

4. Add the chicken back to the skillet and pour in the sauce, which should sizzle and start to bubble. Allow it to bubble and thicken, another 2-3 minutes, stirring frequently. Serve stir fry on top of rice.

5. I used Noble Made from The New Primal for coconut aminos, found at whole foods. See the post for a coconut amino substitute.

6. Coconut aminos are sweeter than soy sauce, and much less salty. They need to be balanced with the toasted sesame oil and a little bit of sodium. No added sugar is needed. Taste the sauce and use these to adjust to your liking.

7. Use a smooth, drippy tahini

8. Serve with rice or cauliflower rice. For low carb, replace the carrots with more squash.

9. Make this vegan or vegetarian by replacing the chicken with 2-3 cups of more vegetables.

23. Instant Pot Buffalo Chicken

Prep Time: 20 Minutes

Cook Time: 10 Minutes

Servings: 4

Ingredients

- 1 ½ pounds boneless, skinless chicken breasts
- ½ cup vegetable or chicken broth
- ½ cup hot sauce (Frank's Red Hot recommended)
- 1 teaspoon garlic powder
- 2 tablespoons butter, ghee, or pressed oil spread
- 1 green onion (optional)
- salt and pepper to taste

Instructions

1. Add all of the ingredients except the green onion to the Instant Pot, cover, and turn vent to closed. Hit "Pressure Cook" for 8 minutes. If you have huge, thick chicken breasts, cook for 9-10 minutes. Allow a natural release for 10-15 minutes, not opening the

vent and leaving the lid on. Then turn the vent to allow any excess pressure to release and open the lid. Watch your fingers during this process, the steam will be very hot.

2. Remove the chicken with a slotted spoon and shred with two forks or with a kitchen mixer on low. Meanwhile, reduce the sauce by turning the instant pot to "sauté" and letting it boil for about 5 minutes. If you'd like a thicker sauce, whisk in 1-2 teaspoons cornstarch till smooth. But don't worry that it's thin, the sauce will coat the chicken well once you combine the two.

3. Mix the chicken with the sauce, stirring well to fully coat. Top with green onion, if desired. Taste and adjust any seasonings.

24. Ground Beef Nachos Supreme

Prep Time: 20 Minutes

Cook Time: 10 Minutes

Servings: 4

Ingredients

Seasoned Ground Beef:

- 1 pound ground beef
- 1 tablespoon chili powder
- 2 teaspoons cumin
- 1 teaspoon smoked paprika
- ½ teaspoon garlic powder
- ¼ teaspoon kosher salt
- ⅓ cup water
- ½ cup fresh or frozen corn

Nachos:

- ½ 12oz bag tortilla chips
- ½ pound good quality American cheese, shredded
- ½ cup low-sodium canned black beans

- 4 green onions, chopped
- ¼ cup chopped cilantro
- ½ cup sliced peppers (sweet mini peppers for mild, jalapeño for hot)
- 2 radish, sliced

Instructions

1. Preheat the oven to 375 degrees F. Add ground beef to a large pan over medium high heat and begin to cook till no longer pink about 5-6 minutes, breaking it up into small bits. Once cooked through, drain any excess fat and add the spices, stirring over medium heat till well-combined. Add ⅓ cup of water and bring to a simmer, until almost all the water has cooked off. Mix corn with the beef to defrost, or cook separately in the same pan once the beef is removed.

2. Cover a large sheet pan with parchment paper. Place the tortilla chips on top, then sprinkle with shredded American cheese. Layer the ground beef, beans, and corn. Bake for about 7-8 minutes until the cheese has melted.

3. Add the fresh toppings - cilantro, peppers, green onions, radish, and any sauces and serve immediately!

4. Good quality American cheese is usually found in "block" form from the deli counter. Ask them to cut you a big piece so you can grate it on a cheese grater. If you can only find Horizon, tear into smaller pieces or remove the individual wrappers and smush them together to grate.

5. For a faux sour cream, blend cottage cheese in a food processor and leave dollops on top of the nachos after baking.

25. Cajun Salmon Pasta

Prep Time: 10 Minutes

Cook Time: 15 Minutes

Servings: 4

Ingredients

- 12 oz pasta (I used linguine)
- olive oil spray or about 1 tablespoon of olive oil
- 4 4-6oz salmon fillets
- 2 large garlic cloves, minced
- 1 cup low sodium vegetable broth
- 1 teaspoon paprika
- ½ teaspoon smoked paprika
- ¼ teaspoon oregano
- ¼ teaspoon cayenne pepper
- salt and pepper to taste
- ⅓ cup heavy cream
- 2 ounces cream cheese

Instructions

1. Start by boiling the pasta in salted water, according to package directions. Drain the pasta, but retain about 1 cup of the pasta water for the sauce. Pat salmon fillets dry with a paper towel, and season with salt and pepper.

2. Meanwhile in a large, non-stick or carbon steel pan, spray olive oil and turn to medium hight heat. Once warmed, add the seasoned salmon, skin side up, and turn the heat down to medium. Sear for 4-5 minutes and don't touch it! The salmon will release naturally from the pan when it's got a nice brown sear. Flip and cook another 3-4 minutes for medium doneness, or until cooked to your liking. Remove salmon from pan and set aside.

3. If there's a lot of excess oil, drain it out of the pan or wipe with a paper towel, but there should just be enough to sauté the garlic on medium low heat, stirring frequently so it does not burn. Add in broth and spices, whisking till combined. Turn heat up to bring to a boil, reducing the broth by about half over 3-4 minutes. Turn the heat back down to medium low and whisk in heavy cream. Simmer till the sauce has thickened - about 2-3 minutes,

stirring often. Stir in cream cheese on low heat till smooth and creamy.

4. Add in cooked pasta, tossing till well-coated over low heat, then add about ⅓-1/2 cup pasta water to thin out the sauce a little bit, if needed. If the sauce is too thin, simmer over medium low heat with the pasta in the sauce - just for 1-2 minutes. Season with salt and pepper to taste.

5. Use defrosted or fresh salmon fillets that have been pat dry. Season at the last second before searing. Salting the salmon early and letting it sit draws out moisture which you don't want before searing. Also don't touch the salmon when searing, it will release from the pan naturally when ready - usually within 3-5 minutes. Moving it around the pan won't give you that nice, brown crust.

6. Use a cream cheese and heavy cream without carrageenan.

7. Salmon can be substituted with shrimp, halibut, cod or scallops for this recipe.

8. To make this low carb, and using the salmon and sauce on top.

9. Nutritional information is for one large serving of pasta (about 3oz per person) and 6oz of salmon.

26. Shrimp Scampi without Wine

Prep Time: 20 Minutes

Cook Time: 25 Minutes

Servings: 4

Ingredients

- ¼ cup olive oil
- 1½ lbs white jumbo shrimp, peeled and deveined
- 10 cloves garlic, peeled and sliced thin lengthwise
- ½ cup vegetable broth
- 1 tablespoon lemon juice *can be substituted with 2 teaspoons distilled white vinegar
- 1 tablespoon butter, chilled
- ¼ cup chopped Italian parsley
- salt and black pepper to taste

Instructions

1. Heat 1 tablespoon olive oil over medium heat in a large cast iron or non-stick skillet until hot. Add peeled and deveined shrimp, lightly salt and pepper

the shrimp, and fry about 2-4 minutes until opaque and cooked through, flipping halfway. Remove shrimp from the skillet and set aside.

2. To the same skillet, add the remaining 3 tablespoons of olive oil. Add sliced garlic and cook about 2 minutes over medium heat, stirring often so it doesn't get dark brown or burn. Once the garlic has softened and become fragrant add vegetable broth, turning heat to high till boiling. Reduce the broth by about ½ it's amount - it will begin to thicken a bit into a sauce after about 1-2 minutes.

3. Turn the heat to low and whisk in lemon juice and butter till smooth. Stir in the cooked shrimp until well-coated. Taste and adjust with salt and pepper.

4. Sprinkle with parsley and serve warm with crusty bread or one of the suggestions in the post..

5. This recipe is a part of my reintroduction series. Lemon is not allowed in the initial elimination phase. It can easily be omitted from the recipe, but I recommend adding some acidity with vinegar or about ½ teaspoon sumac.

6. Lightly salt the shrimp when cooking, and taste to adjust at the end. I find shrimp naturally more salty, so like to leave it to personal preference.

7. To make the original chili garlic shrimp recipe, sauté 1 sliced red jalapeño pepper along with the garlic cloves. Also add 2 more tablespoons of chilled butter at the end.

27. Fish Tostadas (Baja-Style)

Prep Time: 27 Minutes

Cook Time: 15 Minutes

Servings: 4

Ingredients

Baja Fish:

- 1 pound firm, white fish like cod, halibut, mahi mahi, or on ono
- 1 teaspoon garlic powder
- ½ teaspoon paprika
- ½ teaspoon chili powder
- ¼ teaspoon ground sumac
- 1 tablespoon flour (use white rice flour for gluten free)
- ½ teaspoon kosher salt
- 5 corn or flour tortillas
- high heat oil like canola or avocado

Toppings:

- 1 large mango, diced

- ⅓ cup radish, diced

- ¼ cup cilantro, chopped

- finely shredded cabbage or coleslaw mix

Spicy Mayo

- 2-3 tbsp mayonnaise

- 2 teaspoons sriracha or hot sauce

Instructions

1. Preheat oven to 450 degrees F. Spread the tortillas on a large baking sheet and brush or spray them with olive oil on both sides. Bake for 4-5 minutes and flip them, then baking another 4-5 minutes until golden brown. Remove from oven and cool - they should crisp up more as they cool.

2. Cut fish across the filet, about ½ inch thick. In a small bowl, add spices with flour and toss fish strips to coat. Prepare a large plate with paper towels to drain your fish.

3. Chop mango, cilantro, and radish for toppings. Stir together mayo and sriracha in another small bowl. Mix the spicy mayo into the coleslaw mix or

keep them separate and just drizzle on top of the tostada.

4. In a large frying pan, add enough high heat oil to just cover the bottom of your pan. Heat oil over medium high until shimmering. A flick of water that sizzles can tell you if it's ready. Add fish strips and fry for 2-3 minutes until golden brown. Flip and cook another 2-3 minutes. Drain on paper towels.

5. Top crispy tostadas with a little bit of slaw or cabbage, fish, toppings, and then drizzle with spicy mayo.

6. If grilling, omit the white rice flour and sprinkle seasoning mixture directly on the fish fillet. Preheat grill to 425-450 degrees F and cook approximately 8 minutes for a 1 pound fish filet.

28. Healthy Beef Enchiladas

Prep Time: 5 Minutes

Cook Time: 30 Minutes

Servings: 4

Ingredients

Red Enchilada Sauce:

- 3 tablespoons all purpose flour or cornstarch
- 3 tablespoons olive oil
- 1 tablespoon chili powder
- 1 teaspoon smoked paprika
- 1 teaspoon cumin
- ½ teaspoon garlic powder
- 2 cups vegetable broth
- salt and black pepper to taste

Enchiladas:

- 1 pound ground beef
- 1 olive oil spray
- 1 large shallot, chopped (about ⅓ cup)
- 10-12 oz fresh spinach or arugula

- 6 or more corn or flour tortillas I used Central Market's fresh flour tortillas. Tortillaland has good ones as well. Look in the refrigerated sections of grocery stores

Optional toppings:

- cilantro, ¼ cup goat cheese or cream cheese

Instructions

1. Preheat oven to 400 degrees Fahrenheit. Begin by making the sauce - whisk together the flour and oil in a small pot over medium heat. It will become very light golden brown as it bubbles. Then whisk in spices till smooth. Continue whisking for a little less than a minute till fragrant, then pour in the broth little by little till the sauce becomes smooth. Turn the heat to medium high and begin to simmer for about 5-7 minutes till thickened enough to coat a spoon. It will continue to thicken as it cools.

2. Add ground beef to a large pan over medium high heat and cook till no pink remains - about 5 minutes. Season with salt and pepper. Add shallots

and sauté about 1 more minute. Then add spinach or arugula and wilt slightly, about 2 minutes.

3. Spray a 9x13 inch baking dish with olive oil. Pour ¼ cup of the enchilada sauce in the bottom, tilting the dish to make sure it covers the whole bottom. Spoon the beef mixture into the tortillas. You may need more than 6 depending on the size of them. Roll them tightly and place seam side down in the pan. Once all have been placed in the pan, pour the remaining sauce over the top, avoiding the edges of the tortillas.

4. Bake uncovered on the middle rack for 20 minutes. If the top is not brown enough to your liking, you can bake on the top rack another 3-5 minutes.

5. Remove the enchiladas from the oven and allow to rest for a few minutes, adding cheese and cilantro as desired.

6. Recipe calculated using lean ground beef and large flour tortillas. 7-8 WW points.

7. The enchilada sauce can be made ahead and will keep in the fridge for up to 5 days.

8. These healthy enchiladas will work with chicken, turkey, or beef.

9. Old tortillas or ones that have been stored in the fridge have a tendency to crack, especially corn ones! To avoid this, try to buy them fresh and use them within a day of purchasing. If this isn't possible, I wrap them in a wet paper towel and microwave in 15 second intervals till warm and pliable. This should help with the rolling process. At the end of the day, don't worry if they crack - they'll still be delicious and the sauce hides a lot of it!

29. Pan Seared Sea Bass

Prep Time: 5 Minutes

Cook Time: 15 Minutes

Servings: 4

Ingredients

- 1 ¾ pounds Chilean Sea Bass, cut into 4 filets
- salt and black pepper
- 1 tablespoon olive oil
- 1 tablespoon butter
- ¼ cup white wine or vegetable broth
- 1 shallot, chopped small
- 10 oz fresh cherry tomatoes or mini heirloom tomatoes
- 1 tablespoon parsley, chopped

Instructions

1. Take the sea bass filets out of the fridge 10-15 minutes before you begin and pat dry. Season with kosher salt and black pepper on both sides. Preheat

oven to 425 degrees F if using filets thicker than 1 ½ inches.

2. In an oven safe frying pan, heat butter and olive oil over medium-high heat until butter is bubbling, but not smoking/burning. Add sea bass filets flesh side down and DON'T TOUCH THEM for 5 minutes. If it's cooking too quickly, turn down the heat to medium. If you move them around when they're not ready, they will stick to the pan.

3. Once a golden brown crust has formed, flip to skin side down. Deglaze the pan with wine or broth, add chopped shallots and tomatoes. Using a wooden spoon, stir them around the fish without moving the fish. Spoon some of the sauce over the sea bass as it cooks and pan sear for another 4-5 minutes.

4. For a very thick filet (like the ones I used), transfer the whole pan to the oven and bake for 4-7 minutes until fish has cooked through. Serve warm over mashed cauliflower or potatoes.

30. Salmon

Prep Time: 5 Minutes

Cook Time: 15 Minutes

Servings: 4

Ingredients

- 2 tablespoons butter or olive oil
- 4 garlic cloves, minced
- 16 medium-sized raw shrimp, peeled and deveined with tails removed, chopped into ½" pieces
- 4-5 oz cream cheese
- 1 large handful of fresh spinach leaves (roughly 1 cup)
- ¼ teaspoon Primal Kitchen New Bae seasoning*
- 4 center cut salmon filets, 4-6oz per person
- ¼ cup panko breadcrumbs
- salt and black pepper
- Parsley for garnish, if desired

Instructions

1. Preheat oven to 400 degrees Fahrenheit (200 C). In a large pan, melt butter or olive oil over medium heat. Add minced garlic cloves, stirring often, till soft and fragrant (but not brown), about 1 minute. Stir in chopped shrimp and cook, stirring often, till just opaque - about 2-3 minutes. Turn off the heat and mix in cream cheese and spinach, till everything is well-coated, then add the New Bae seasoning. Taste and adjust any seasonings.

2. Arrange salmon fillets skin side down on parchment or on a sheet pan sprayed with oil. Pat dry. Make a small ½" slit down the center and pull apart to stuff the shrimp mixture in. Season filet with salt and pepper, then spoon the mixture into the slit, allowing it to spill out a bit on the top.

3. Top with panko and bake at 400F for 15-18 minutes for medium cooked fillets. Panko should be lightly brown on top. Sprinkle parsley for garnish, if desired.

www.ingramcontent.com/pod-product-compliance
Lightning Source LLC
Chambersburg PA
CBHW070956250726
48663CB00002B/246